*God's Pathway
to Healing*

HERBS THAT HEAL

God's Pathway to Healing

HERBS THAT HEAL

by

Reginald B. Cherry, M.D.

ALBURY PUBLISHING
Tulsa, Oklahoma

Note: The directions given in this book are in no way to be considered a substitute for consultation with your own physician.

2nd Printing

God's Pathway to Healing: Herbs that Heal
ISBN 1-57778-135-X
Copyright © 1999 by Reginald B. Cherry, M.D.
Reginald B. Cherry Ministries, Inc.
P. O. Box 27711
Houston, Texas 77227-7711

Published by ALBURY PUBLISHING
P. O. Box 470406
Tulsa, Oklahoma 74147-0406

CONTENTS

Introduction

1 God Has a *Pathway to Healing* for You 19

2 God's Pathway to Herbs that Heal 51
    Anxiety, Insomnia, Stress 61
    Arthritis 67
    Asthma 72
    Congestive Heart Failure 73
    Depression 76
    Diabetes 79
    Dizziness, Ringing in the Ears 79
    Fatigue 80
    Fibrocystic Breast Disease 81
    Headaches (Migraines) 83
    Hepatitis and Liver Damage 85
    High Cholesterol, Blood Pressure Problems . . 87
    Hot Flashes (Menopause), PMS 92
    Immune System (Colds, Infections) 94
    Irritable Bowel Syndrome (Spastic Colon) . . . 98
    Memory 100
    Prostate 101
    Skin Rashes, Eczema, Psoriasis 104

3 Good Nutrition for Overall Good Health . . . 125

4 Praying With Understanding
   for Your Pathway 135

5 Your Next Steps in God's *Pathway to Healing* . 149

Reginald B. Cherry, M. D.
   A Medical Doctor's Testimony 153

About the Author 157

Resources Available Through
   Reginald B. Cherry Ministries, Inc. 159

Become a *Pathway to Healing* Partner 163

INTRODUCTION

Linda and I have a great concern for our family — the body of Christ. We want to protect believers from confusing medical half-truths by giving you sound information. The devil can and does distort and twist information to get us off track.

Many people have taken an interest in herbs these days, yet myths and unknown dangers can keep us from realizing their many benefits. Notwithstanding the poor or incorrect information, the healing power of herbs has generated an intense interest in the United States, as well as in Europe and many other countries. We want to separate the myths from the facts for you concerning the most common herbs in this minibook.

We use many names to refer to herbs: botanicals, nutraceuticals, and herbal medicine. Herbal medicine, herbal treatments, and the purchase of herbal products currently amount to an industry of over $1.5 billion annually. Herbs represent the fastest growing area in health food stores and pharmacies now that they have moved into the mainstream medical community. In past centuries, people used herbs as part of medical treatment. Then, modern medicine evolved away from this practice and depended on more synthetic drugs. Today, the pendulum is swinging back the other direction.

For the first time ever, insurance companies are approving and paying for herbs as medicines if physicians prescribe them. For example, American Western Life Insurance

Company and Blue Cross of Washington and Alaska recently announced new health plans that cover the cost of herbal medicines prescribed by health practitioners. In times past that would never have happened. This illustrates the potency we are beginning to see in some of these plant-based products. A big insurance company paying for herbal preparations? It makes us stop and think, *Could there be something to this?* Yes, there is.

Doctors still do not learn about herbs in medical school. I've had to research this topic myself because medical professors don't teach much about herbs. However, changes are just around the corner. Let's review what happened a few years ago. A major conference took place between several proponents of the herbal industry and the U.S. Food and Drug Administration

(FDA). The FDA astounded those representing the herbal industry by saying, "We need some good treatments that are not addictive to help people sleep. We need new medicines for migraines that work and won't have side effects. We need things that can help people's memory that we don't have in traditional medicine."

Very conservative by nature, the FDA administrators usually require a ten-year, $200,000 study before they accept a new form of treatment. Now they're saying, "Look, we're open to the use of herbs." Insurance companies are saying, "We'll pay for it." There's got to be something to all this. Many of you may say, "This is all new to me." I was trained in one of the best medical schools in the nation, the University of Texas Medical School in San

Antonio, Texas, and wasn't taught anything about herbs, either.

When I read the literature and see the studies, there's so much that herbal medicine can do. But think of this carefully: If plants contain chemicals that can help us, we must also be aware that plants can contain chemicals powerful enough to harm us. We've got to get good information because there are some herbs we should avoid.

Also, we might be tempted to think that plants cannot be as effective as prescription medicines, but 40 percent of our prescription medicines come from the plant kingdom. A lot of people have heard of some of these drugs. Some of them, such as morphine and other various painkillers, come from the opium poppy plant. Other drugs used for years in cancer treatment come from a periwinkle plant. None of this is particularly new information to those who research medicine. For example, there is a little chemical in willow bark called salicin, which is the basis of aspirin. Aspirin is a simple product used by billions worldwide to cut the risk of heart attacks, stroke, and possibly even colon cancer. These examples demonstrate that there is a great precedence for looking to God's plant kingdom for help.

Numerous studies have proven that many herbs have a significantly positive effect. European scientists have made studies of these plants available for several years. We will be covering many of these herbs individually. For example, two herbs that are showing strong benefits are feverfew and ginkgo biloba. Feverfew can stop migraine headaches by affecting the dilation and constriction of the blood vessels in the brain. Ginkgo improves blood circulation in the brain and can have a positive effect on decreasing ringing in the ears. Ginkgo can also help with headaches and memory loss. Scientists are now proving that many plants have genuine medical benefits.

Using herbs requires certain precautions. The United States doesn't regulate herbs the way it does traditional medicines. We currently face two challenges with herbs: 1) we don't have any way to guarantee their purity, 2) we don't have a way to regulate their potency. There are about 600 herbal preparations available in the United States, which vary in quality and purity. Some medicinal herbs may cause allergic reactions in susceptible individuals, and others may not be right to use for particular health conditions. We don't want to start taking herbs randomly without knowing their benefits and potential side effects.

We also know certain plants are deadly. The ancient philosopher Socrates committed suicide using the tea of hemlock, a common plant. Because of the potential dangers, many herbal retailers have taken herbs such as comfrey, colt's foot, pennyroyal, and borage off the shelves. Many of these dangerous herbs have toxins that can destroy the liver because of an alkaloid chemical in them. A few years ago in the Southwest, a common herb called chaparral caused a woman some severe problems. She had been taking one or two capsules daily for ten months and then increased it to six capsules daily. She was supposedly using it for arthritis, but it damaged some of her vital organs, eventually requiring a liver and a kidney transplant. Good information could have prevented this tragedy.

On the other hand, we don't want to refuse the plants God has provided to help with illness. At a recent medical conference, a medical school professor who is also a physician gave a presentation on herbal medicine, plants, and the various chemicals they contain. The doctors attending this conference had very little knowledge about herbs, but the professor had factual information to demonstrate their value. Since he was on the faculty of a well-known medical school, the doctors respected him and listened carefully to what he had to say. What we saw at this conference is a great example of how the truth about herbs is just beginning to spread.

With an incredible explosion of good information, God is revealing to the medical world His original plan to take care of His sons and daughters through His plant kingdom. Traditional medicine is only now recognizing the value of the information we are making available in this minibook. For the first time, some doctors are beginning to understand that herbs can help heal their patients. It takes a while for doctors to be open to nontraditional medicine, but this minibook may help open the door to discussing herbal treatments with your doctor. The information in this book should not be used as a substitute for advice from a qualified health-care practitioner.

God has a *Pathway to Healing* for you and part of that pathway may involve using natural herbal medicine. You'll see just how wonderfully He has provided for us in the plant world. Praise God!

Chapter 1

GOD HAS A *PATHWAY OF HEALING* FOR YOU

Chapter 1

GOD HAS A *PATHWAY OF HEALING* FOR YOU

Since Linda and I began teaching about God's *Pathway to Healing* on our television program, we've been getting letters full of wonderful praise reports from people who have been healed by God in various ways. In each case, God touched them when they had little hope of healing. What is exciting about these letters is not just that God heals people today, but that He heals them in various ways that minister to each person's individual situation. In many cases the people who write us had to give up their own ideas about how God would manifest their healing. Some had to follow His leading concerning certain medicines or dietary changes. Others had to face some spiritual issues that God showed them which held the key to their healing. In so many cases the writers of these praise reports had to submit to God's direction and follow His *Pathway to Healing* for their lives.

I was at a medical conference when a physician came up to me and said, "Dr. Cherry, you've got to hear this story." She told me about a woman who had a malignant lump in her breast. She gave the woman a copy of my book, *The Bible Cure,* which the woman read. The woman then had her church begin to pray for her according to the specific ways taught in the book. She went back for a second biopsy before surgery and the doctor could find no trace of the cancer. She was totally healed. Thank God!

She had found her *Pathway to Healing* through the intercession of her church (we will discuss how she began praying in chapter four). We have taught this concept of different pathways to our patients for years. What's your way? Well, you have a unique way that will bring about a manifestation of healing to your body ordained and divinely appointed by your Father.

The problem is that we think that all healings should be the same and that they should all be instantaneous the moment we pray. Yet, all healing is supernatural in the sense that Jesus took our infirmities and bore our sicknesses (see Matthew 8:17). But sometimes healing is a process that involves the natural. If God has directed a person to a natural substance or a natural process, that substance or process is anointed by Him and it is no less supernatural! In our focus upon methods that we insist God must follow, we forget that people are getting healed in so many various ways. It is all to the glory of God.

Let us show you what we mean. One television viewer wrote to us about how God used natural measures to heal him. God anointed natural substances to manifest his healing. He wrote, "I was watching you on television recently, and you spoke about God's *Pathway to Healing*. I found that pathway in taking natural vitamins and herbs, but I wouldn't have known it if I hadn't first listened to you." He explained in his letter,

You see, I suffered a heart attack because my artery was 85 percent closed due to high cholesterol. I had to have a stent put in the artery, and, praise the Lord; the doctor did a wonderful job. Everything was fine and is still fine today. However, my doctor put me on a certain medication, and I asked him, "What are the side effects?" This is what he said, "You may develop a liver or kidney problem later on down the road, but we will deal with that when the time comes. For now we need to get your cholesterol down at any cost," which was 286 at the time of the heart attack.

Well, first of all I didn't like what he had to say about the side effects and who would? I told him that I had read Dr. Cherry's book and that I was going to pray about it and see what God had to say to me about this medicine. So I prayed.

He told us that he read his Bible and received his spiritual prescription. He went on to say, "I got the vitamins and herbs that you mentioned in the book, and the last time I had my cholesterol checked it was down significantly. I still have to get it lower, but I'm working on it."

Because he did it God's way under the leading of the Holy Spirit, he's not going to face liver or kidney problems down the road. Having the stent put in will be the last time he has to worry about his heart. (A stent is made of an inert material, usually stainless steel, with a self-expanding mesh introduced into the coronary artery to keep it open.) Do you see how his healing was still God-given even though he used vitamins and herbs? Through obedience to God's direction, a natural substance contributed to a supernatural healing!

What he shared in his letter shows God's perfect timing for his life. He first started learning about God's *Pathway to Healing* in 1996 through our television program. However, we didn't teach about the plant he needed until early summer, 1999. He needed to know about hawthorn. Hawthorn is an herb that keeps your heart strong. When someone has a stent put in an artery, the heart needs to be strong. He had learned in 1996 that God has distinct and unique ways to manifest healing. Now he knew he needed to pray about whether hawthorn and Co Q-10 (a supplement we had previously discussed on television) were part of his *Pathway to Healing*.

This man's testimony tempts us to go out and do exactly what he did to get our healing to manifest. Or, when we hear about a new herb or supplement the temptation is to go out and purchase it, hoping that we will be healed through taking it. However, in both cases that would be the wrong thing to do. We wouldn't want anyone to use hawthorn or Co Q-10 without praying. It might not be what God planned as their *Pathway to Healing*.

Please don't just accept all the information we share with you as being God's final word on the issue and start taking herbs we've discussed. Though the information is dependable, it may be right for one believer but not for another. God may call that person to use something else. In every case when we present information on our programs or in our minibooks, we want our viewers and readers to pray about whether this information is something God wants them to use. God knows exactly what you need as an individual. And He will reveal it to you. He promises that.

Jesus said, "And I will ask the Father, and he will give you another Counselor to be with you forever — the Spirit of truth" (John 14:16-17 NIV). One of the purposes of the Holy Spirit is to lead us into all truth, even medical truth. Before Jesus left His disciples, He told them that when the Holy Spirit came He would "tell you what is yet to come" (John 16:13 NIV). The Holy Spirit knows what will and what won't manifest healing for us. Our job in this minibook is to give you information that the Holy Spirit can use to guide you down your unique pathway.

Each person has to allow God to choose the *Pathway to Healing*. The letters our viewers send often show us many different ways in which God can lead a person to a manifestation of their healing. One testimony from a viewer demonstrates why just taking an herb is a bad idea. God may be leading you down a completely different pathway. We love this praise report because many people need to know that what someone harbors in their heart may be causing the manifestation of illness in their body. This person wrote,

> I just saw your program on television, and Linda spoke about how your letters encourage others. I know there are many different pathways of healing and one of them is the power of forgiveness. Let me explain, I used to have ulcerative colitis. I had it for over three years. I went to my doctor and he flat out told me that it wasn't cancer yet, but that it was serious.

She shared that every day for those three years, when she would have a bowel movement, she would pass a lot of blood. The colitis made her feel she had to go to the bathroom every hour. One evening she began to cry when she was praying. She wrote,

I poured my heart out to the Lord and asked Him to show me what was blocking the healing of this colitis. With my eyes closed tightly, pleading to the Lord, I saw His beautiful face. He was smiling, and I heard Him say in my spirit, "You have to forgive."

I answered, "Lord, I don't know what You mean. Who do I have to forgive and for what?" Still smiling at me, my mind was flooded with names. Yes, people who had somehow hurt me in the past came flashing back now. Funny, I thought I put those hurts out of my mind. Every time I would see that person I would say hello and even give them a hug, yet deep inside I still felt the sting of the hurt.

So right then and there I asked the Lord to forgive me for my unforgiveness. I forgave those who had hurt me, but I felt led of the Lord to do one more thing. The next day I called each of those people, and I asked them to forgive me because I had been holding a grudge against them and I told them that I forgave them too. That whole day I didn't use the bathroom once, and when I finally did, praise the Lord, there was no blood.

Then she announced:

And to this day, five years later, there is no sign of colitis. Yes, my *Pathway to Healing* at that time was forgiveness. Isn't God just wonderful?

Some believers don't realize that harboring things like unforgiveness inside throws the entire body off balance. For example, ulcerative colitis is due to an imbalance in the immune system that causes the body to attack the lining of the colon and the intestinal area. Inflammation then occurs. For this person unforgiveness threw her immune system off. It is hard for anyone to serve God and finish the race that is set before them in that shape. Yet a person with an illness caused by unforgiveness might try all kinds of treatments to bring about a healing without addressing the true cause of their illness. Linda and I can't emphasize enough the importance of asking God's guidance about your healing with a mind open to hearing whatever He may direct you to do.

These wonderful praise reports show what can happen when people begin understanding that their pathway is unique. The

Bible supports this, saying that we are "fearfully and wonderfully made" (Psalm 139:14). As you pray and understand just how unique God has made you, you will find your pathway. Your pathway may involve a natural substance, forgiveness, or another area that God will reveal to you.

Our quest to understand the process of healing can often frustrate and confuse us. Why? Well, Jesus explained that we have an enemy in this world who is out "to steal, and to kill, and to destroy" us (John 10:10). That enemy is not as interested in attacking our physical bodies as much as in hindering the anointing that is contained within our physical bodies. He also tries to hinder our understanding of God's process for healing. That's why praying before we use herbs and medicines is so important. We want the Holy Spirit to clear away the misconceptions and point out our unique *Pathway to Healing*.

Think about it. If you are sick, you will be distracted from doing the things that God has called you to do. Christians have a great deal of spiritual power from the Holy Spirit, and they can rock the world with their obedience to God's call. Second Corinthians 4:7 says, "But we have this treasure in earthen vessels, that the excellency of the power may be of God, and not of us." This treasure, the anointing power of God, resides within us. It is that anointing which the enemy is intent on trying to cripple and weaken by hurting our bodies. However, we can take heart. That very anointing also empowers us to victory and to finding our *Pathway to Healing*.

Understanding the finished work of Jesus' sacrifice is a first step to finding that pathway. One of the first things we like to point out to patients is that the blood of Jesus is a finished work and so is our healing. Jesus already healed us 2,000 years ago. First Peter 2:24 supports that principle of healing by saying that Jesus, "by whose stripes ye were healed," has *already* healed us. Since we were healed 2,000 years ago, we actually seek and believe God for the *manifestation* of that already-accomplished healing in our bodies. It may seem like a minor point, but when you begin asking God to illuminate the pathway that will lead to the manifestation of an already-accomplished healing in your body, you are "rightly dividing the word" (2 Timothy 2:15). You acknowledge to God the real meaning of that incredible sacrifice He made. God placed our disease and infirmity upon the body of His own precious Son. Jesus bore in His body not only our sins, but also our diseases that result from that sin. With this understanding you then have bold confidence to pray for His guidance to your *Pathway to Healing*.

The next principle we want you to understand relates to the different pathways. We've shown you in present-day testimonies how God uses various ways to heal. Now let's explore two different healings recorded during Jesus' ministry. We want you to consider Mark 10:46-52 and John 9:1-7. The revelations contained in these two healings performed by Jesus literally changed the way Linda and I practice medicine. It will change the way you pray and your expectations concerning the kinds of answers God will give to your prayers.

In these two scriptures we see two men, each with the same disease (blindness), each having an encounter with Jesus, and each being totally healed. However, from the time of their encounter with Jesus until healing was manifested in their bodies, we see a totally different set of circumstances.

As we examine these two healings, we want you to understand that there is a unique pathway to your healing and from the symptoms of potentially serious diseases. God never intended nor willed for you to suffer sickness in your body. So be encouraged as we discover God's healing pathway for you.

SUPERNATURAL HEALING MAY BE A PROCESS

Many of the healings of Jesus occurred instantly, supernaturally, and dramatically.

At other times, healing took some time through a process. In Luke 17:14 the ten lepers were healed "as they went." Jesus didn't heal them as they stood there. He told them to show themselves to the priest, which they had to do in order to be declared clean. They still had leprosy as they stood there listening to Jesus tell them what to do. They still had leprosy as they turned to leave; but as they made their way to the priest something wonderful happened — God healed their leprosy. Yet even in this supernatural event, God anointed the process of their obeying Jesus' command and healed them *after* they had left Jesus.

In the case of Bartimaeus in Mark 10:46-52, we see two important principles at work even when healing is instantaneous:

1. Jesus asked Bartimaeus to *express his faith that the Lord can and will heal.* In His encounter with Bartimaeus, Jesus knew his affliction. Nevertheless, He asked him, "What wilt thou that I should do unto thee?" He asked Bartimaeus this question in order to get the blind man to show his faith by telling Jesus, "that I might receive my sight" (v. 51).

2. In asking what Bartimaeus wanted, Jesus required that he *speak to the mountain of his afflictions.* By that we mean that Bartimaeus spoke directly to the problem — his blindness — and expressed his faith that the Lord would heal his blindness. Bartimaeus' faith in addressing the affliction directly made him whole. He received an immediate and complete manifestation of his healing from blindness.

YOUR PATHWAY TO HEALING MAY INVOLVE ANOINTED NATURAL MEANS

Let's compare the healing of Bartimaeus with what is perhaps one of the most unusual healings (of blindness) recorded in Jesus' ministry (see John 9:1-7). This healing gives us a unique revelation from the Word of God and explains why we need to let God choose our pathway.

Remember that this man had the same disease as Bartimaeus; that is, he was blind. When Jesus touched him and anointed his eyes with a mixture of mud and saliva, interestingly, healing did *not* manifest instantly. In fact, Jesus gave the command, "Go, wash in the pool of Siloam" (v. 7). This command involved a series of actions that would require the blind man to go down a pathway, reach down into the pool called Siloam, place water in his hands, and wash his eyes. That one command was really a set of instructions, but God anointed those actions and the natural substances that Jesus used. The healing occurred through natural substances, yes, but it was still a supernatural healing because God anointed those substances.

Why, of all the healings Jesus performed, did God include this incident in the Bible? The key part of this account is found in John 9:7 where it states, "He went his way therefore, and washed, and came seeing." We believe it illustrates two important revelations about healing:

1. *The manifestation of your healing may involve you first following a set of instructions.*

2. *As you are obedient to the leading of the Holy Spirit and "go your way," you will be healed.*

This brings up a common point that arises in the letters from people who watch our program: "Aren't we supposed to be healed by faith?" Yes, we know our faith heals us. It's simply that sometimes the faith we have in God's anointing flows through another mechanism along with the supernatural. Perhaps His anointing will flow through the hands of another human being. Sometimes His anointing flows through a medicine, an herb, a natural treatment, or a supplement, but that makes it like what happened in John 9 to the blind man. Jesus touched him with mud and saliva, and he wasn't healed immediately. He was healed as he obeyed a set of instructions that Jesus gave him.

He told him to find the path, walk down to the pool called Siloam, reach down in the pool, and wash the mud and saliva off his eyes.

As he went his way he was healed, John 9:7 states. It's still faith and it's still a supernatural healing. Linda and I have noticed that there's a lot of condemnation in the body of Christ regarding healing. Believers tell other believers who receive their healing after medical treatment, "Well, you just didn't have enough faith. You had to go to the doctor." They may even condemn you for taking a medication, a natural supplement, or having surgery. However, this isn't how God sees it.

Notice that Jesus didn't condemn that blind man in John 9. He healed him just as fully as He healed Bartimaeus in Mark 10 of the identical disease. Jesus said, "Bartimaeus, your faith made you whole." He was healed through supernatural means alone, but the blind man in John 9 was just as healed by *supernaturally anointed* natural substances.

Listen to this carefully — the blind man in John 9 had the opportunity to say, "Wait a minute, Jesus, Bartimaeus was healed through supernatural means alone. What's this mud and saliva thing? Don't You have the power to touch me, anoint me, and heal me?" But the blind man didn't ask that because he had faith in the Healer. He was obedient and the healing anointing flowed through the means that God had chosen.

You, too, have a way. It might be an immediate healing through faith. Thank

God, if it is! Who in the world wouldn't want to be healed like Bartimaeus? But for many of us, it's a combination of natural medicine and God's supernatural anointing. God asks us to do what we can do in the natural realm; then He does what we can't do in the supernatural realm. Our healing is a matter of faith and a matter of God's intervention. The point is you have a unique pathway to the manifestation of your own healing. That's the good news. Amen? Amen!

That is why God instructed Linda and me to teach people His principles concerning His *Pathway to Healing*. We see in John 9 that healing anointing can flow through natural substances; that is, substances we can touch, taste, and feel. In this case, the healing anointing from Jesus flowed through mud and saliva.

As we study the Bible, we see from Genesis to Revelation the emphasis that God has placed on natural substances and that He uses them to bring about the manifestation of our healing. We see how plants, certain animals, and even the leaves of trees (see Revelation 22:2) were used as part of the *Pathway to Healing* for people. God is still in the healing business today. He created us and knows the best method to use for us to be healed.

As we reflect on the healings that God illustrates in Mark 10 and John 9, we can petition Him to reveal to each of us our unique *Pathway to Healing* through the leading of the Holy Spirit — the One who guides us into all truth and shows us things to come (see John 16:13). We can do this with a mind and heart open to what God tells us. In the healings we have seen with our patients, often God's *Pathway to Healing* for them involves a combination of both reliance on supernatural intervention and the use of natural substances. We then encourage them to share their healing manifestation with others. To share what God has done for us is the same as praising Him. Sharing how God manifests our healing builds up the faith of others and helps encourage them. Our God is no respecter of persons — if it happened for us, it can happen for them. We receive letters from people who write about their *Pathway to Healing*. We regard these letters as praise reports of what God is doing to help people find their unique pathway. Linda and I share the letters on our program to stir up our viewers' faith and to help other people overcome their illnesses by finding His *Pathway to Healing* for them.

By understanding these two illustrations from Jesus' ministry and seeking God for our *Pathway to Healing,* we can understand that we are not limiting God. Instead, we are being totally open in our petitions to Him by acknowledging Him as our supernatural Healer. We also acknowledge that He provided natural ways through which healing anointing may flow. Then, as we tell others about what God has done, God receives glory and others learn what they can do to receive His provision for their own *Pathway to Healing.*

YOU HAVE A PATHWAY TO HEALING

For some of us, learning that God does not intend for us to be sick constitutes an important step on our *Pathway to Healing.* For others, a mature understanding of what the finished work of Jesus means gives the needed boost to their faith. However, lately Linda and I have seen that an openness to letting God be the One who chooses the *Pathway to Healing* has caused major breakthroughs in the lives of so many of our patients and viewers. We rejoice with them in the glory that goes to God for each of these healings.

As we explain the specific ways God has provided to prevent illness and to deal with the symptoms of illness through herbal medicines, think of the different ways that Jesus healed the two blind men. Remember that the healing doesn't come through the herbs. However, if God chooses an herb for your pathway, He will anoint that herb to work for you by His power.

Chapter 2

GOD'S PATHWAY TO HERBS THAT HEAL

Chapter 2

GOD'S PATHWAY TO
HERBS THAT HEAL

First a Word . . .

Linda wonders about all the things that we find in capsules when we see the shelves of herbs and supplements in stores today. She once said teasingly, "Pretty soon we're just going to have all these little capsules around the plate and no food."

I don't think it will get that far. All those supplements might make it seem as though we don't have to eat anymore, but think about why we're seeing so many herbs and supplements. I think it is because we're in the last days. Jesus talked about the wars and rumors of wars, but He also mentioned pestilence that would come in the last days.

We're seeing the ozone layer thin. With every breath in and out, our immune system takes a hit and undergoes certain amounts of weakening because of pollution, particularly if you live in the city. We're seeing strange infections. We read about epidemics such as various salmonella and e-coli infections that affect the colon and cause food poisoning in thousands of people. As we see more and more pestilence, we need a strong immune system. Because of these dangers, God is showing us how to fortify our immune system and protect ourselves in these last days. That's a significant reason we see the explosion of herbal medicines and food supplements in capsule form. Many doctors who used to feel that eating well was enough have begun recommending that their patients take nutritional supplements. Soon herbs will be on their list as well.

A lot of information on herbs comes to us from new scientific studies. At the medical conference we mentioned earlier, doctors sat in amazement as they heard evidence that supported herbs' potency in treatments for many diseases. Many of them didn't believe that herbs could be helpful until a professor showed them careful scientific studies that proved just how effective some herbal treatments could be. They began to understand that the doctor of the future is going to have to combine traditional medicine with knowledge of natural supplements. If we can, we'd rather use natural herbs instead of the prescription medicines. If we must use a prescription medicine, we should remember that half of those also came from plants. God has been inspiring scientists for many years to discover substances in our world that can help us. And really, it makes sense that He would do that. From the very beginning when God gave people plants to eat for food, He has pointed to the plant world for the sustenance of life: "Behold, I have given you every herb bearing seed, which is upon the face of all the earth, and every tree, in the which is the fruit of a tree yielding seed; to you it shall be for meat" (Genesis 1:29). And later, God tied His healing anointing on natural substances we use for food to our submission to Him. He also gave detailed instructions on diet:

"And ye shall serve the Lord your God, and he shall bless thy bread, and thy water; and I will take sickness away from the midst of thee" (Exodus 23:25). God has never ceased to be interested in our health and has even provided our prescription medicines through His generous inspiration. In many cases, however, His original provision of medicinal plants has fewer side effects and works more effectively for many conditions.

WHAT IS AN HERBAL MEDICATION?

An herb is a plant whose flowers, leaves, or roots contain chemicals that have a potent effect on the human body for healing. We hear various terms these days which refer to herbal medicines — nutraceuticals, botanicals, herbal remedies — but the bottom line is that God provided certain plants with chemicals in them that can act in the human body to promote healing under His direction.

Herb [L. herba, grass]

A plant with a soft stem containing little wood, esp. an aromatic plant used in medicine or seasoning. The plant usually produces seeds and then dies down at the end of the growing season.

Tabers Cyclopedic Medical Dictionary 1997

We talked about salicin from willow bark as a mild pain reliever and anti-inflammatory medicine. It is interesting that using the herb from willow bark does not cause the stomach problems that man-made aspirin does. This herb is familiar, but the herbs that follow may surprise you, such as celery or cinnamon. The fact that ordinary substances like these have healing properties is a testimony to God's faithfulness in providing for our healing from the very beginning of creation.

Since we are still just learning how much help lies beneath the stems and leaves of the plant world, many herbal medications are not standardized in America. That's why it's hard for Linda and me to give you exact doses. We all have to be careful about that. We found this out with garlic. We bought some garlic pills that required taking several to get the amount equivalent to one garlic clove. Another company required only one garlic pill for that same dosage. Manufacturers have, however, agreed upon standardized dosages for many other herbs and supplements.

You can simply read the label and follow the recommended dosage.

Herbs are potent and it is very important to understand proper dosages. That means you need to tell your doctor that you are taking herbs and/or supplements if he is treating you for an illness or disease. Medicines and herbs can interact. For example, a woman took ginkgo with a medication her doctor prescribed after bypass surgery. She had a hemorrhage in her brain because both the ginkgo and the prescribed medication affected the blood platelets.

The challenge is to learn which herbs really work and which ones are safe. Doctors have to sift through a great deal of new information frequently. Something new comes out almost every day, and we must evaluate what is accurate. That is the purpose of this minibook.

Even though herbs are proving themselves to be very beneficial because of the
new scientific data that supports their
effectiveness, doctors are not usually open
to recommending them. The use of herbs
was rare until a few years ago. Traditional
medicine has been even slower to adopt
the use of these natural plant treatments.
Now herbs are being presented in medical
school lectures. Doctors were taught years
ago that if it wasn't written on a prescription pad, you shouldn't use it. Then scientists discovered that plain aspirin, which
comes from the bark of a willow tree, in a
low dose of 81 mg., could help protect
people from heart disease and blood clots.
We are tempted to think that more is
better or that faster is better. Sometimes
the mild dosages that herbs provide are a
sign of God's wisdom. Yes, times have

changed a great deal in medicine. It's an exciting time, yet herbs can hold hidden dangers in prescribing them to patients.

That's one reason doctors were at the medical conference I mentioned earlier. They wanted to learn all they could about herbs. Their patients are taking them, but they don't always realize that they need to tell their doctors what herbs they are taking. Doctors learned at the conference that they need to know about drug inter-actions with herbs and potential side effects their patients might experience. You need to know this too. We've tried to make it easy for you. There are charts at the end of this chapter on side effects and on common drug interactions with herbs. For your protection, you should tell your doctor if you are taking herbs.

In the following herb entries we mention the dosage of the herb when available. Dosage information is provided as a general guideline. In some cases, however, the optimal dosages are still being determined. Some herbs are not standardized and should be taken according to the package label directions.

Which Herb for What?
Anxiety, Insomnia, Stress

Kava-kava

Kava-kava is a natural herb from a pepper plant found throughout the South Pacific islands from Hawaii to New Guinea. It has sometimes been called God's natural tranquilizer. If you are going through a stressful time in your life, kava-kava can be used instead of calling your doctor to get a prescription for *Valium, Xanax,* or one of the other prescription tranquilizers. Kava-kava can also be used with valerian for sleep, but when used alone it helps people relax during the day. Be sure to read the directions on the label. It is available in capsule form, without a prescription. It is natural and safe if used properly.

You can overdo anything, and kava-kava is no exception. If you take too much of this substance, you can get too groggy and you will want to sleep all the time. You can, however, use a higher dosage at night. It is safe if you use it as it was intended for stressful periods. As with anything, we must follow the instructions and not assume that more is better.

When you read the following warnings, you begin to realize that herbs can contain very potent chemicals. Don't let that scare you. Taken at the recommended doses for *occasional* anxiety or sleeplessness, kava-kava can help. The proper dosage is safe.

Caution: Kava-kava has side effects such as gastrointestinal problems or allergic skin reactions in a few people. If it is used for a prolonged period of time it can cause a scaly rash and eye irritation. If it is used in excess of the recommended amount, it can make you dizzy. Side effects of long-term use include temporary yellow discoloration of the skin, hair, and nails.[1] While it helps with anxiety, it can be dangerous if you are depressed. Avoid taking if you are pregnant or nursing. Because of its apparent sedative action, this herb should

---

[1] Ann Ronan, MA, and Dennis deLeon, M.D. "Kava for the Treatment of Anxiety." *Clinical Reviews of Leading Herbal Therapies.* Ed. John La Puma, M.D., Atlanta: American Health Consultants, 1999, 45.

not be taken when operating machinery or vehicles.

Kava-kava also causes problems in patients with Parkinson's disease. It can make the disease worse. Patients who take medications such as *Xanax, Tagamet,* or *Hytrin* can become lethargic and confused after combining kava-kava with them. Kava-kava should not be used with benzo-diazepines, barbiturates, antipsychotics, or alcohol. Avoid exposure to the sun while taking this herb; it can trigger an immune reaction.[2]

Valerian

What a problem sleeping has become today! Doctors are seeing more and more

---

[2] Melanie Johns Cupp, Phar M.D. "Herbal Remedies: Adverse Effects and Drug Interactions." *American Family Physician,* 59 (March 1999): 1243.

patients who complain of difficulties with sleeping. We receive many letters asking about herbs to help with sleeping problems. Valerian is one herb that has received a great deal of attention in medical journals. It is a very common herb and is available without a prescription. It is a mild sedative that is not habit-forming while most prescription sedative preparations are. Valerian is number eight on the world's list of best-selling and most purchased herbs. Why do we tell you that? Because that statistic tells you it works. People don't buy items that don't work for them.

You can remember Valerian very well because it tastes bad and smells like dirty, stinky socks. If you can get it down, it will relax you and give you a good night's sleep. Perhaps the bad smell might stimulate you a little bit. No, it really does work. The commonly used dosage is 900 to 1,200 milligrams for sleep at night. It should be taken about forty-five minutes before you are ready to go to sleep. In other words, give it some time to work. You may need to wait an hour after eating a large meal for it to absorb in your system. This herb definitely works, and it is very helpful. You can take valerian and kava-kava together if the valerian alone is not strong enough to help you sleep.

Caution: You should be very careful not to drive or use heavy machinery when you take this herb. The effect of taking very large doses is unpleasant and chronic use may result in headaches, giddiness, insomnia, arrhythmias, spasm, hallucinations, excitability, and dependence. It is important to realize that valerian potentiates other sleeping pills and will make them stronger.[3] It should not be used with them unless guided by professional judgment. No side effects are associated with occasional use.

ARTHRITIS

Evening Primrose Oil — EPO

Evening primrose oil (EPO) has proven to be very beneficial in the treatment of arthritis. Herbs such as celery, feverfew (usually used for headaches), willow, and devil's claw have also brought relief to arthritis patients by functioning as anti-inflammatories. Other supplements that act

---

[3] Dominion Herbal College (Canada). "Herb of the Month, Valerian: From the Chartered Herbalist Course Materials." Webpage. Updated: 3 April 1999. Accessed: 31 August 1999. http://www.dominion-herbal.com/herb_month/Valerian.htm.

as anti-inflammatory agents are glucosamine and omega-3 fatty acids. Chondroitin sulfate also helps arthritis by providing moisture to the joints. In many cases, combining EPO with the above mentioned herbs and/or supplements has proven very effective in easing arthritis symptoms. EPO should be taken according to label directions. EPO has proven helpful with other health problems such as eczema, fibrocystic breast disease, and premenstrual syndrome (PMS) which will be covered later in this minibook.

Caution: Evening primrose oil can cause seizures if used with certain medications such as phenothiazines or with certain epileptic drugs.[4] Rarely, it can cause abdominal discomfort, nausea, and headaches.[5]

---

[4] Victor S. Sierpina, M.D. "Top Twenty Herbs for Primary Care." Unpublished Paper, May 1999: 4.

[5] "Table 3. Herbal Therapy Primer." *Primary Care Special Edition* 3:1 (1999): 20a.

Ginger

The same spice we loved in gingerbread as children has proven to be good therapy for many ailments. In capsule form, ginger has been used for circulatory problems, dizziness, nausea, indigestion, and ringing in the ears. It has been used with success for motion sickness. It has been used for migraine headaches because it affects chemicals that cause inflammation and affect platelets. This multi-purpose herb is also being used extensively for arthritis, including rheumatoid arthritis, because of the anti-inflammatory properties of ginger. Remarkably, ginger has hardly any side effects! This is an herb that requires reading the label for the proper dose.

Caution: Rarely, people have gotten mouth ulcers from using ginger. Ginger should be taken under the care of a physician when taking anticoagulants or anti-inflammatory drugs, even aspirin. This is very important. This herb can interact with these drugs and cause serious problems with hemorrhaging. Patients with gall bladder disease should avoid taking ginger. Very high doses of ginger could cause gastrointestinal upset or stomach ulcers.[6]

Horseradish

Would you think horseradish could fight various forms of arthritis? Most of us think it could open up our nasal passage, but not help with arthritis! There are chemicals in horseradish that have a strong effect on arthritis. If you feel that

---

[6] Susan K. Hadley and Judith J. Petry. "Medicinal Herbs: A Primer for Primary Care." *Hospital Practice* (15 June 1999): 115.

this herb is part of your *Pathway to Healing,* take as directed on package label.

Licorice

For some people, licorice has become a very effective herbal preparation for arthritis. An anti-inflammatory ingredient in licorice has an effect similar to hydro-cortisone and other corticosteroid hormones as it is broken down in the body. Research has shown that it also can be used to treat chronic hepatitis and liver cirrhosis. It is sometimes used as a diuretic to reduce fluid retention. In addition, licorice contains isoflavones that can help with menopause symptoms. However, licorice is best used occasionally. Take as directed on package label.

Caution: Don't take this herb if you have kidney disease (kidney insufficiency), hypertension, heart disease, or problems with potassium levels. It should not be taken while taking diuretics. Side effects with high doses or long-term use are loss of potassium and high blood pressure. Some people have gotten headaches from using licorice. You will need to read the label for the proper dosage. We always encourage prayer to receive peace that this herb is one God has designated for you.

ASTHMA

Onions

Herb companies are making it easy to take almost every herbal preparation. Onions are now available in extract form. Onions can be helpful with breathing difficulties because the chemical they release relaxes the smooth muscle lining of the bronchial tree. This allows more air to enter the lungs. It is very interesting that a well-known food has such wonderful medical properties. If using onion extract, see package directions.

CONGESTIVE HEART FAILURE — CHF

Hawthorn

God has provided some potent, naturally occurring chemicals in a plant known as hawthorn. It provides protection against congestive heart failure. Congestive heart failure (CHF) allows fluid to build up in the lungs and the lower extremities. The heart also enlarges. It's a devastating disease because it's a slow death. Fluid accumulates in the body, and you can literally suffocate to death. It's a major problem, but thank God He has provided great help in this area.

Hawthorn was God's original ACE drug. Scientists thought *they* had discovered the original inhibitor of this angiotensin-converting enzyme; ACE, as we call it. However, God had already made a provision for heart disease in His creation. If you have been diagnosed with CHF, you may be on a prescription ACE drug such as *Vasotec, Zestril, Accupril,* or *Cozaar.* There are many of them. They can save your life, but hawthorn can still be useful.

Hawthorn has also been used with digitalis. *Lanoxin* is one of the trade names for digitalis, which comes from the foxglove plant. Digitalis was one of the first strong heart medications available.

CHF is one form of heart disease that is increasing while other forms have decreased slightly. Hawthorn has been shown to increase blood flow through the heart. In CHF, hawthorn strengthens the heart muscle contraction in conjunction with prescription medications such as ACE inhibitors. In other words, it will help improve the circulation by strengthening the heart muscle.

There is a substance that can be combined with hawthorn. That substance is Co Q-10. It is not an herb. It is an antioxidant manufactured in the human body that is also found in plants. A dosage of between 90 and 200 milligrams daily of Co Q-10 has been used for treating congestive heart failure. This antioxidant seems to significantly strengthen the heart muscle by improving the pumping ability of the heart muscle. We can combine Co Q-10 with God's natural ACE inhibitor, the hawthorn berry. Both come in capsule form.

Yes, this is an herb you can combine with prescription drugs. If you were to take hawthorn with an ACE drug, the dosage of the prescription may need to be lowered since hawthorn is a natural ACE inhibitor. Praise God, you can even experience the manifestation of healing of congestive heart failure. As you do what you can do in the natural realm, God will do what you can't do in the supernatural realm. He provided this herb as an incredible help in the healing process for CHF.

Caution: This drug has no adverse side effects and no known drug interactions.

DEPRESSION

St. John's Wort

Many people are becoming familiar with St. John's Wort. *Wort* is an English word for plant. In Germany St. John's Wort is the number one prescribed anti-depressant. This herb is used for various mental conditions that stem from chemical imbalances. Research shows that it has a significantly positive effect on some types of depression, mostly the chronic mild forms. It can also alleviate anxiety. Extracts standardized to 0.3 percent of active ingredient (hypericin) are taken in dosages of 300 mg. three times a day in capsule form. St. John's Wort has been helpful for insomnia by taking 900 mg. one hour before bedtime. There is also a liquid extract that can be used to make a tea. Follow the instructions on the package to make the tea.

Caution: St. John's Wort is generally used for mild to moderate depression. If someone is suicidal or has severe depression, St. John's

Wort may not be enough. It can also react with certain medicines known as selective serotonin re-uptake inhibitors (SSRI's) such as *Paxil, Prozac,* and *Zoloft.* If you are on a medication for depression, you need to talk to your doctor to find out if it will react with St. John's Wort. Generally, doctors are not recommending that you mix St. John's Wort with any other medication for depression.

Rare side effects are dry mouth, dizziness, gastrointestinal complaints (constipation), and confusion. In addition, avoid sunlight and UV light treatments if using St. John's Wort. This herb causes some people to become sensitive to light causing sunburn.[7]

---

[7] Mady Hornig, M.D. "Hypericum (St. John's Wort) for Treatment of Depression." *Clinical Reviews of Leading Herbal Therapies.* Atlanta: American Health Consultants, 1999, 9.

DIABETES

Cinnamon

Common cinnamon, the spice we associate with baked goods, is proving to stabilize blood sugar in diabetes. The incidence of diabetes is increasing rapidly. We've mentioned the use of chromium picolinate (800-1000 mcg. daily) for diabetes on our television program. We've read letters from viewers who were able to stop using insulin after this supplement dramatically lowered their blood sugar level. God has provided another blood sugar lowering substance: cinnamon. Cinnamon now comes in a standardized dosage in capsule form. Follow the label instructions for dosage recommendations.

DIZZINESS, RINGING IN THE EARS

Ginger (see Ginger entry under Arthritis).

Feverfew (see Feverfew entry under Headaches).

FATIGUE

Ginseng

Ginseng has been recommended often for increasing physical stamina, mental capacity, and to relieve stress. Frankly, research data is lacking on ginseng. Most reports are stories of people who feel better when they take it. Physicians need solid research. More studies examining ginseng are now in progress.

Ginseng can be taken as an herb, be used in cooking, or used as a tea. Brands of ginseng vary. If you are fatigued and would like to find out if ginseng is helpful for you, read package labeling carefully. Look for label instructions showing the standardized percentage of ginsenosides, the active ingredient. The ginsenoside content should be over 10 percent. Package labeling will recommend specific dosages for desired use (capsule, tea, food additive, etc.).

Caution: If you are on *Warfarin*, avoid ginseng. Prolonged use at high doses may cause high blood pressure, insomnia, uterine bleeding, and sore breasts in women. Avoid taking ginseng during pregnancy. Avoid ginseng herb mixtures — some are contaminated with germanium.[8]

FIBROCYSTIC BREAST DISEASE

Evening Primrose Oil — EPO

Evening Primrose Oil (EPO) works well for women with fibrocystic breast disease.

---

[8] Schiedermayer, M.D. "Ginseng for the Improvement of Constitutional Symptoms." *Clinical Reviews of Leading Herbal Therapies.* Atlanta: American Health Consultants, 1999, 26.

This disease is demonstrated by very thick, fibrous tissue in the breasts and tends to increase the risk of breast cancer. Fibrocystic breasts can be determined by a mammogram. However, if you have fibrocystic breast disease, steps can be taken to slow down this disease and may help with discomfort. Taking 400-800 I.U. of "natural" vitamin E daily, discontinuing the use of caffeine, and consuming EPO have all proven to be very beneficial. EPO should be taken according to label directions.

Caution: Evening primrose oil can cause seizures if used with certain medications such as phenothiazines or with certain epileptic drugs.[9] Rarely, it can cause abdominal discomfort, nausea, and headaches.[10]

---

[9] Sierpina, M.D., 4.

[10] "Herbal Therapy Primer," 20a.

HEADACHES (MIGRAINES)

Feverfew

Linda read a letter on our program that shared a praise report about feverfew:

My husband and I watch your program, "The Doctor and the Word" faithfully every week and have learned so much. I had the worst headaches a day or two before my menstrual cycle would begin and they lasted several days. Sometimes I would get another headache right after my cycle was over. I just felt terrible, but I took Dr. Cherry's advice and bought some feverfew herb that was combined with white willow. It really and truly works. I didn't have a headache at my last cycle. I started taking them again around my next cycle, and everything worked normally. I didn't have a headache then either. Thank you so much for your love for people. I can see that you both honestly care and want to help people as much as you can by seeking God's direction.

We have received many other tremendous praise reports from people who have been on feverfew.

Feverfew is used primarily to treat and prevent headache problems. It is a very strong herbal medication, and I do mean *medication.* It's an herb, but it acts in the body like a medicine. It has a strong effect on the blood vessels and the inflammatory response around the blood vessels. Feverfew is less commonly used for dizziness, ringing in the ears, and for women who have had menstrual irregularities. This herb is best known for its effects on headaches.

Caution: Feverfew should not be used during pregnancy because it stimulates the uterus. Avoid using during nursing after pregnancy. If you are trying to prevent headaches, use it for four to six weeks in accordance with package directions.[11]

HEPATITIS AND LIVER DAMAGE

Licorice (see Licorice entry under Arthritis).

Milk Thistle

Milk thistle is a plant, now available in capsule form, which can be very effective in treating hepatitis C. It can protect liver function and help restore function in livers that have been damaged by hepatitis. Many hepatitis patients have been prescribed interferon, which is the medical world's treatment for this disease. Half of the patients do not respond to interferon.

---

[11] Sierpina, M.D., 4.

In six to twelve months, half of the patients that *seem* to respond experience a relapse. Interferon is very expensive and has side effects.

Cirrhosis is another liver problem for which traditional medicine offers no solution. Cirrhosis is scarring of the liver. Milk thistle has an active ingredient, silymarin, which can help reverse this damage. Silymarin contains a mixture of flavonoid derivatives, which work directly on the liver cells. It can be used to reverse both cirrhosis and chemical damage in the liver. Milk thistle should be taken according to package label directions.

Consider the case of an alcoholic who turns their life around by giving their heart to Jesus. Their liver may be damaged because of the effects of alcohol. But, God is a restorer. He can supernaturally restore their liver, but He may also guide them to use milk thistle in combination with their supernatural trust in Him.

Caution: Milk thistle can act as a mild laxative. Loose stools may occur during the first few days of use.

HIGH CHOLESTEROL, BLOOD PRESSURE PROBLEMS

Celery

God created a plant that lowers blood pressure and cholesterol. It is celery. Celery has been prescribed in Asian cultures since 200 BC. The Asian people consumed half-pound amounts every week for health benefits. A study in America showed that after consuming two large stalks of celery daily, there was a 12-14 percent drop in systolic blood pressure readings. These same participants dropped their cholesterol by seven points. If you need to lower your cholesterol or your blood pressure, you can either eat two stalks of celery daily or take celery in extract or capsule form. Follow package directions for proper dosage.

Caution: There are no known side effects by the intake of celery.

Garlic

Garlic has proven to have multiple benefits. It contains over 30 different cancer-protective and cancer-fighting chemicals. It thins the blood. It lowers blood pressure. It increases the level of HDL (the good) cholesterol. Scientists have also discovered that it functions as a mild antibiotic. It has a killing effect on certain types of bacteria.

If you eat raw garlic you may have noticed that it presents certain social problems. The odor from garlic is carried on your breath, in your sweat, and in every pore of your skin. There is a way to alleviate this problem. Garlic is now available in an odorless supplement form. Linda and I take two garlic capsules daily, equivalent to one clove of garlic. Some brands require more for the same equivalency. Read the label carefully making certain you are taking a dose equal to one clove.

"Well," you may wonder, "what about sautéing it and putting it in foods?" You may do this. The problem with cooking garlic is that it is changed chemically. It is not as offensive socially if it is cooked, but it is not as medically beneficial. Here is one theory: If garlic is not offensive to people close to you, then it is not offensive to tumor cells, high blood pressure, or elevated cholesterol.

You wouldn't think that something as common as garlic would need a warning, would you? However, garlic thins the blood and affects blood platelets. It would be wise to discuss taking garlic with your doctor if you are on prescription medication.

Caution: Garlic should not be taken if you are on anti-inflammatory drugs or Coumadin. You should stop taking garlic before surgery.[12] Some surgical patients have had trouble with bleeding when they did not stop taking garlic prior to their surgery.

---

[12] Hadley, et al. 109, 112.

Rosemary (for low blood pressure)

Rosemary is often used in cooking but it can also serve other purposes. It is often used for people with low blood pressure *and* it acts as an appetite stimulant. We don't mention much about people who are fighting a problem with low body weight, but we receive many letters asking about this problem. Many people find it difficult to eat. They don't have an appetite for one reason or another. Some people are fighting certain diseases in their body and their appetites are suppressed. In those cases, rosemary can be a stimulant to the appetite. It is available in capsule form or it may be consumed in food. The advantage of capsules is that it can be taken in a measured amount every day, which keeps the blood level constant. Follow label instructions for recommended daily dosage.

HOT FLASHES (MENOPAUSE), PMS

Licorice (see Licorice entry under Arthritis).

Black Cohosh

Black cohosh has shown very positive results in treating women with symptoms of perimenopause and menopause. Symptoms may include hot flashes, sleep disturbances, headaches, irritability, and depressive moods. Women under the age of forty who have hormonal problems or who have had a hysterectomy, have had successful benefits from taking this supplement. The standardized dose is equivalent to 40 mg. root extract taken two times daily. Treatment is required for at least eight weeks to alleviate symptoms.

Juvenile menstrual disorders and premenstrual syndrome (PMS) patients have found relief by taking black cohosh extract. Take this herb according to package label instructions.

Caution: If dosages are taken in excess of recommendations, some women have experienced gastric irritation.

Evening Primrose Oil — EPO

Evening primrose oil (EPO) has also been used to alleviate the symptoms of premenstrual syndrome (PMS). Some researchers believe that the omega-3 fatty acids in this herb add a missing substance whose absence causes PMS. EPO should be taken according to label directions.

Caution: Evening primrose oil can cause seizures if used with certain medications such as phenothiazines or with certain epileptic drugs.[13] Rarely, it can cause abdominal discomfort, nausea, and headaches.[14]

---

[13] Sierpina, M.D., 4.

[14] "Herbal Therapy Primer," 20a.

IMMUNE SYSTEM
(CANCER, COLDS, AND INFECTIONS)

Astragalus

Astragalus is a plant used in China for centuries. Strong clinical evidence indicates that astragalus is successful as an immune-stimulating, immune-restoring substance. It has a protective effect against colds, flu, viruses, and cancer cells. Astragalus extract increases natural killer cells.

Dosages vary depending on the form of Astragalus (dried root, liquid, or extract). Like most herbs, this is available over the counter. Take this supplement according to package label directions.

Caution: Astragalus should not be used in acute illnesses where fever and thirst are present.

Echinacea

Echinacea is one of the most popular herbs on the market today. Native Americans found this wildflower, also known as purple coneflower, to be very beneficial in treating colds, flu, and infections. Echinacea stimulates the immune system causing resistance to upper respiratory tract infections, acts as an anti-inflammatory for rheumatoid arthritis, and can hasten wound healing, if used topically. Echinacea stimulates white blood cells to attack viruses and various bacteria as it increases the lymphocyte production.

Rather than being used continuously, echinacea should be used as needed at the *onset of symptoms* or in the early stages of infection. It should not be taken continuously longer than six weeks, followed by a resting period of at least three weeks before taking this supplement again. The human body builds a tolerance against echinacea and it will no longer work effectively in fighting our illnesses. Echinacea is known as "nature's antibiotic." Echinacea is packaged in various forms: capsule, liquid, and topical preparation. It should be used according to package label directions.

Caution: In rare cases nausea and diarrhea have occurred while taking echinacea. Avoid echinacea during pregnancy. People with autoimmune disease or kidney problems should not use echinacea.[15]

Garlic (see Garlic entry under High Cholesterol and Blood Pressure Problems).

Goldenseal

Goldenseal has also been called one of "nature's antibiotics." This American herb is often combined with echinacea in capsule form. It is used for colds, viral infections, bacterial infections, and digestive

---

[15] "Herbal Therapy Primer," 209.

tract problems. Goldenseal also has anti-inflammatory properties. It has even been used to help shrink the prostate in men. Goldenseal is becoming rare because it has been harvested in its wild natural environment. It should be taken according to recommended package directions.

Caution: Goldenseal should not be used for prolonged periods.[16] It should not be combined with goldenthread or Oregon grape, which have berberine in them. Avoid taking if you are pregnant or nursing. Persons with a history of hypertension should avoid this herb. Large dosages or frequent use cause nausea and dizziness in some people.

---

[16] Dónal P. O'Mathúna, Ph.D. "Goldenseal: The Golden Cure for Common Colds?" Clinical Reviews of Leading Herbal Therapies. Atlanta: American Health Consultants, 1999, 21.

Shitake Mushrooms

The Shitake mushroom is immune boosting and cholesterol lowering. It also fights active cancer cells. Shitake mushrooms are available in health food stores and grocery stores. This is a natural food and you may eat any amount you desire.

Caution: Certain varieties of mushrooms are poisonous. Make certain you know the variety you are consuming. Mushrooms should not be picked and eaten in the wild unless you are an *expert* on mushroom species.

IRRITABLE BOWEL SYNDROME (SPASTIC COLON)

Peppermint

Peppermint was originally used after a full meal to relax the sphincter between the esophagus and the stomach. It has recently been shown to help with irritable bowel syndrome (IBS). IBS is a condition of alternating diarrhea and constipation, bloating in the abdomen, and gas. This was previously referred to as spastic colon. The natural ingredient in peppermint capsules (not candy) is an antispasmodic. It relaxes the colon and helps relieve symptoms. Peppermint should be taken in a coated capsule form because it passes through the stomach and works to relax the colon. Peppermint has also been used for nausea, headaches, and insomnia.

Caution: People with gastroesophageal reflux, gallbladder problems, or liver disease should not take peppermint.[17]

---

[17] Hadley, et al., 121.

MEMORY

Ginkgo Biloba

Ginkgo biloba has shown good results in helping with memory and circulation. In Europe doctors have been using it for the cerebral area to increase circulation and blood flow to the brain. It can also be used for circulation in other parts of the body, such as the lower extremities. Ginkgo also helps with tinnitus, vertigo, and headaches. An article was written in *JAMA, Journal of the American Medical Association,* about ginkgo's preventive effect against Alzheimer's disease. In patients diagnosed with this disease, ginkgo has proven to slow down the rate of development. Take according to package label directions.

Caution: Ginkgo should not be used if you are taking aspirin, *Coumadin,* anti-inflammatory, or anticoagulant drugs.

PROSTATE

Goldenseal (see Goldenseal entry under Immune System).

Saw Palmetto

Saw palmetto (*serenoa*) is the fruit of a small shrub in the palm family native throughout Florida, where it is wild-harvested. Saw palmetto has become known as a natural treatment for symptoms of an enlarged prostate, also known as benign prostatic hyperplasia (BPH). It has been proven to be as effective at shrinking the prostate in men as a prescription medication.

Surgery was the main treatment for prostate enlargement even a few years ago. Fortunately, medical science has reached far beyond this option. Saw palmetto is effective because it inhibits the enzyme 5-alpha reductase. It contains the same chemical as Proscar, an expensive prescription medication. Proscar can cost as much as $2.00 per day while saw palmetto can cost as little as 20 cents per day. If you suffer from BPH, this condition can often be dealt with by taking this herb in a standard dose of 160 mg. twice daily.

Caution: Men over fifty should have regular yearly prostate examinations. Saw palmetto treats only BPH. If a more serious condition exists, a consultation with your physician is necessary. Rarely, stomach cramping has occurred while taking saw palmetto.

Pygeum

Scientists have now discovered that extracts from a plant called pygeum can have a similar beneficial effect to saw palmetto on the prostate gland. The bark from this African tree contains beta-sitosterol, a chemical that reduces inflammation, swelling and edema (fluid accumulation) in the prostate gland. In addition, many studies indicate significant improvements in patients with various urinary tract problems. Extracts from pygeum bark have been shown to be as effective as prescription medications. When men do not get the relief they need from saw palmetto alone, we often combine it with pygeum. Combining these two herbs gives added anti-inflammatory benefits that reduce the prostate.

Pygeum, taken in a dose of 100 mg., can significantly increase urinary flow. This can prevent men from having to get up to urinate many times during the night (nocturia). Patients have had very few side effects from taking this treatment. Pygeum extract can be taken in a dose of 100-200 mg. daily, divided into two doses. A combination of saw palmetto and pygeum is available in supplement form, which is very convenient.

Caution: Rarely, mild stomach or gastrointestinal problems occur.

Skin Rashes, Eczema, and Psoriasis

Aloe Vera

If any herb claims to be America's number one folk remedy, it is aloe vera. The aloe vera plant originally comes from eastern and southern Africa. Aloe vera is listed as an ingredient in many lotions and even in facial tissue. Research has shown that aloe vera gel placed on a wound causes it to heal more quickly. It is recommended for minor burns, sunburns, and rashes. Some surprising research demonstrated a significant improvement in people suffering with psoriasis when aloe vera gel was applied three to five times daily as a topical treatment.[18]

Caution: Aloe vera is a very potent plant. When taken internally, it can increase menstrual bleeding, cause diarrhea, and upset electrolyte balance. *Never* take it if you have a suspected intestinal obstruction, inflammatory bowel disease, or during pregnancy.[19]

Evening Primrose Oil — EPO

Interesting, EPO in an oil form has been used to treat eczema. Eczema is a problem with chronic inflammation of the skin. This herb has also been used for psoriasis, another chronic skin disease. Traditional medicine's typical solution to psoriasis is

---

[18] Hadley, et al., 106.

[19] Hadley, et al., 109.

to use steroids. However, steroids have some serious side effects. Sometimes God instructs us to use them, but psoriasis has been treated with EPO effectively in many cases. EPO should be taken according to label directions.

Caution: Evening primrose oil can cause seizures if used with certain medications such as phenothiazines or with certain epileptic drugs.[20] Rarely, it can cause abdominal discomfort, nausea, and headaches.[21]

Impatiens

Impatiens is also known as jewelweed. This plant grows wild in Appalachia. Jewelweed has been successfully used topically for skin rashes and poison ivy. Ancient applications required crushing the stems and leaves to extract the juice. They

---

[20] Sierpina, M.D., 4.

[21] "Herbal Therapy Primer," 20a.

would then apply it to the affected skin rash. Fortunately, it is now available in tincture form. Apply it to affected area according to package label directions.

Caution: No side effects or problems are known when used properly.

Uva-Ursi

Bearberry, or *uva-ursi*, is one of the more exotic herbs. Uva-ursi is sometimes used as a diuretic and to aid with urinary tract infections. It is also used as an anti-septic, for skin infections, hemorrhoids, and other aggravating external problems. The tannin in uva-ursi works as an astrin-gent while the allantoin in this herb causes skin to heal faster.[22] This is mostly used as

[22] On Health Network Company, Seattle. "Uva Ursi." On Health: Herbal Index. Webpage. No update date. Accessed: 31 August 1999. *http://onhealthnet workcompany.com/chl/resource/herbs/item, 16066.asp.*

a topical, but uva-ursi is formulated in capsules, tablets, tea, and tinctures.

Caution: High tannin content may produce gastric discomfort is some people. Do not use longer than seven days without consulting a physician.

Side Effects and Warnings for Selected Herbs

Astragalus	Do not use in acute illnesses where fever and thirst are present.
Black Cohosh	Upset stomach. Avoid if pregnant or nursing.[23]
Echinacea	Diminishing effects if used longer than three weeks. Not recommended for more than 10 days for those with compromised kidney function.[24] Avoid during pregnancy.
Ephedra *(ma-huang)* Not recommended!	Hypertension, insomnia, arrhythmia, nervousness, tremor, headache, seizure, cerebrovascular event, myocardial infarction, kidney stones.[25]

Evening Primrose Oil	Abdominal discomfort, nausea, headache, seizures if mixed with phenothiazines. Do not take if you have a history of epilepsy.[26]
Feverfew	Stimulates uterus, avoid if pregnant or nursing. Use caution if you are on anticoagulants.[27]
Garlic	Occasional gastrointestinal distress at first few doses. Possible bleeding if combined with other anticoagulants or anti-inflammatory drugs.[28]
Ginger	Possible bleeding if combined with other anticoagulants.[29] Avoid if gallbladder disease is present.
Ginkgo Biloba	Possible bleeding if combined with anticoagulants. Avoid if taking aspirin, *Coumadin,* anticoagulants or anti-inflammatory drugs.

Ginseng	Do not use in acute infections or in kidney failure. High doses and long-term use can cause hypertension and insomnia, in addition to sore breasts and uterine bleeding for women.[30] Avoid if pregnant or nursing.
Goldenseal	Diminishing effects if used longer than three weeks. Side effects from prolonged use or large doses: nausea, high blood pressure, or dizziness. Avoid if pregnant or nursing.[31]
Kava-kava	Eye irritation. Sedation, difficulty talking and thinking, involuntary muscle movements in the neck or trunk, eyes moving and staying upward, exacerbation of Parkinson's disease.[32]
Licorice	Do not use if you have kidney disease, congestive heart failure, hypertension, problems with potassium levels, or on cardiac medications. Do not take with other diuretics. Avoid use if pregnant or if you have diabetes. Do not use longer than 4-6 weeks. Side effects: loss of potassium, high blood pressure.[33]

Milk thistle	Can act as a mild laxative, possible loose stools.[34]
Peppermint	Can worsen gastroesophageal reflux, gallbladder, or liver disease.[35]
Saw palmetto	Headache, nausea, or dizziness. Possible hypertension.[36]
St. John's Wort	Rare: gastrointestinal disturbances, allergic reactions, fatigue, dizziness, confusion, dry mouth, photosensitivity.[37]
Uva-Ursi	Do not use longer than 7 days without consulting a physician.
Valerian	May impair concentration and/or ability to drive or operate machinery.

---

[23] "Herbal Therapy Primer," 19a.

[24] Ibid, 20a.

[25] Cupp, 1243.

[26] Sierpina, M.D., 4.

[27] Ibid.

[28] Hadley, et al., 112.

[29] Ibid, 115.

[30] "Herbal Therapy Primer," 21a.

[31] O'Mathúna, Ph.D., 21.

[32] Christian Millman. "Natural Disasters." *Men's Health*, (April 1999), 93.

[33] "Herbal Therapy Primer," 21a.

[34] Ibid.

[35] Hadley, et al., 121.

[36] E. P. Barrett, M.D. "Use of Saw Palmetto Extract for Benign Prostatic Hyperplasia." *Clinical Reviews of Leading Herbal Therapies*. Atlanta: American Health Consultants, 1999, 1.

[37] Hornig, M.D., 9.

CAUTION: HERBS CAN BE DANGEROUS

There are a few herbs that can be dangerous and must be used with caution or avoided completely. Think about this for a moment. If there are potent beneficial substances in herbs, there could also be equally potent harmful substances and, in fact, there are. People tend to think that because there is little regulation of herbs in the United States that they must all be safe. Let us discuss some of the herbs that can cause problems.

Chaparral

Though single herbs can be dangerous, the combination of certain herbs together or the combination of herbs with certain prescription medications can also result in severe drug and chemical interactions. For example, garlic, ginkgo, and ginger all have mild blood thinning effects. Though they generally can be taken together in a healthy person, certain people have reacted to this combination in the form of internal hemorrhaging. Again, I emphasize; this is rare but does point out the potency of these various herbs.

Chaparral is a common herb used in the southwestern part of the United States and is known locally as "creosote bush."

Several deaths have been reported with the use of this herb. It causes hepatitis which, in many cases, can advance very rapidly with even low dosages. The damage often occurs so quickly that it becomes irreversible. Do not use chaparral or any herbal mixture containing this compound.

Coltsfoot

Coltsfoot is a flowering plant used in certain herbal cough medicines and teas. This herb also has a chemical in it that can cause liver irritation and damage. It is often mixed with other herbs. You should carefully read the label and avoid any herbal mixture containing coltsfoot.

Comfrey

This herb should be avoided. It has been used to make comfrey teas and traditionally has been taken for gastritis and abdominal discomfort. However, it contains chemical agents that can seriously damage the liver and even lead to liver failure requiring a liver transplant. Avoid taking this herb internally.

Ephedra *(ma-huang)*

Ephedra *(ma-huang)* is a stimulant that some people use to lose weight. *Ma-huang* is a common ingredient in many over-the-counter weight loss products. The problems with this herb arise from its stimulating properties, which means it can significantly elevate blood pressure and heart rate. It can also cause restlessness and difficulty sleeping well at night. Many patients will develop chronic insomnia while using this product. Some dangerous problems have been reported with the herb *ma-huang* because the rise in blood pressure and heart rate is often unpredictable.

In persons who may not be aware of any underlying heart condition, this could become serious and even lead to a heart attack. Palpitations are very common when using *ma-huang,* and patients often report an irregular heartbeat. Please consider carefully before beginning over-the-counter weight loss products, and be led by the Spirit of God. *Ma-huang* is sometimes called the "herbal phen-fen." *Phen-fen* was a prescription medicine combination that had to be taken off the market a few years ago because of its adverse effect on heart valves. *Ma-huang* may help you lose weight, but the price you may pay to achieve your weight loss would not be worth it if you developed a heart attack or a severe blood pressure problem. There are better ways to lose weight, and this is one herb we discourage patients from using.

Sassafras

Sassafras is a root bark from a tree that grows naturally in the eastern portion of North America. Sassafras tea is made from this herb. Sassafras contains a chemical called "safrole" which is a potent cancer causing agent. There is little documentation of any medical value to sassafras. Because of the safrole content, we recommend it be avoided.

Herbs to Avoid

Chaparral

Coltsfoot

Comfrey

Ephedra or *ma-huang*

Sassafras

Possible drug interactions with herbs

Ephedra *(ma-huang)* – caffeine, decongestants, stimulants

Evening Primrose Oil – phenothiazines *(Compazine, Phenergan)*

Garlic – anti-inflammatory drugs or Coumadin

Ginger – aspirin, anticoagulants, or anti-inflammatory drugs

Ginkgo Biloba – aspirin, *Warfarin (Coumadin)*, ticlopidine *(Ticlid)*, clopidogrel *(Plavix)*, dipyridamole *(Persantine)*

Ginseng – *Warfarin (Coumadin)*

Kava-kava – sedatives, sleeping pills, antipsychotics, alcohol, *Xanax, Tagamet,* or *Hytrin,* benzodiazepines (diazepam, lorazepam, *Valium, Ativan*)

St. John's Wort – antidepressants, selective serotonin re-uptake inhibitors (SSRI's) such as *Paxil, Prozac, Zoloft,* and others

Conclusion

When purchasing over-the-counter herbs, other supplements, and health food products, get good factual information. The marketplace is driven today by money. This often becomes more important than sharing accurate information and providing you, the consumer, with products that will help you. A good source of accurate information is a physician or nutritionist who has studied and had experience with more natural therapies using supplements, herbs, and other compounds that complement traditional medicine. In this book, we have taught you how to let the Holy Spirit guide you through prayer and through God's peace so that you can obtain herbs that will allow God's healing anointing to flow through them and help your body. As your Creator, God designed you in a fearful and wonderful way, and He will guide you to the appropriate natural products that will become part of your *Pathway to Healing.*

Remember that all healing is based on faith; faith that we were healed by the blood of the Lamb 2,000 years ago. It is God's desire for us to walk in divine health, and He has shown us endeavors that we must do, both on the supernatural side and the natural side, to see the full manifestation of healing in our bodies.

May you finish the course with joy that God has called you to finish and may your days be long and satisfied according to Psalm 91.

Chapter 3

GOOD NUTRITION
FOR OVERALL
GOOD HEALTH

Chapter 3

GOOD NUTRITION FOR OVERALL GOOD HEALTH

As we have seen, herbs can have a special role in treating a variety of symptoms and illnesses in the human body. They should not be looked at, however, as a substitute for basic underlying good nutritional intake.

For several years, scientists have studied the various diets found around the world. At the top of the list is the Mediterranean diet. Some of the lowest rates of heart disease and cancer recorded in the world have been noted in those countries around the eastern Mediterranean. It is felt that their unusually good health is in large part related to their nutrition. There is a consistency to their dietary intake. I would urge you to study the basic outline of the Mediterranean diet listed below and adopt as many of these principles into your own diet as possible.

THE MEDITERRANEAN DIET

The Mediterranean diet contains many of the food sources rich in the vitamins and minerals needed for consumption. We highly recommend this diet which closely corresponds to Genesis 1:29 and 9:3.

1. **Olive oil.** Replaces most fats, oils, butter, and margarine. Use in salads or

cook with it. Raises level of the good cholesterol (HDL) and may strengthen immune system function. Extra virgin oil is preferable.

2. **Bread.** Consume daily, not sliced white bread or even sliced wheat bread, but either make or buy dark, chewy, crusty loaves.

3. **Pasta, Rice, Couscous, Bulgur, and Potatoes.** Pasta is often served with fresh vegetables and herbs sautéed in olive oil, occasionally with small quantities of lean beef. Dark rice is preferred. Couscous and bulgur are forms of wheat.

4. **Grains.** Alternate cereals such as wheat bran, $1/2$ cup, 4-5 times weekly, and Bran Buds ($1/2$ cup) or oat bran ($1/3$ cup).

5. **Fruit.** Preferably raw, 2-3 pieces daily.

6. **Beans.** Pintos, great northern, navy, kidney, $1/2$ cup, 3-4 times weekly. Bean and lentil soups are very popular (with a small amount of olive oil).

7. **Nuts.** Almonds (10 per day) or walnuts (10 per day) are at the top of the list.

8. **Vegetables.** Dark green vegetables are prominent, especially in salads. Eat at least one of these daily (cabbage, broccoli, cauliflower, turnip greens, or mustard greens) and one of these daily (carrots, spinach, sweet potatoes, cantaloupe, peaches, or apricots).

9. **Cheese and Yogurt.** Unlike milk and milk products, some recent studies indicate cheese may not contribute as much to clogged arteries. In the Mediterranean diet, cheese may be grated on soups or a small wedge may

be combined with a piece of fruit for dessert. Use the reduced-fat varieties (the fat-free often taste like rubber). The best yogurt is fat-free, but not frozen.

You should consume the following foods only a few times weekly:

10. **Fish.** The healthiest are cold water varieties: cod, salmon, and mackerel. Trout is also good. All these are high in omega-3 fatty acids. Salmon is an excellent source of calcium.

11. **Poultry.** Can be eaten 2-3 times weekly. White breast meat is best. Remove skin.

12. **Eggs.** Eat in small amounts 2-3 times weekly.

Consume the following an average of three times per month:

13. **Red Meat.** Use only lean cuts with fat trimmed. Also use in small amounts to "spice up" soup or pasta. The severe restriction of red meat in the Mediterranean diet is a radical departure from the American diet and is a major contributor to the low cancer and heart disease rates in these countries.

Typically, a Mediterranean meal would consist of:

1. **Salad.** Eat with each meal. Fresh greens and other vegetables with olive oil, vinegar, and/or lemon juice.

2. **Soup.** Often with chopped celery, garlic, carrots, onions (sometimes in a chicken stock), with added herbs and a small amount of grated cheese (use low-fat).

3. **Pasta.** A staple of many meals, often made with fresh vegetables and herbs

sautéed in olive oil, occasionally a bit of beef or chicken is added.

4. **Rice.** Prominent in this diet and includes dark rice, pilafs, etc.

5. **Breakfast.** Often dark bread or cereal (such as those mentioned above), a piece of fresh fruit, and perhaps a small amount of yogurt or a slice of cheese.

6. **Tomatoes, Onions, Lemon Juice.** All common in the Mediterranean diet.

Chapter 4

PRAYING WITH UNDERSTANDING FOR YOUR PATHWAY

Chapter 4

PRAYING WITH UNDERSTANDING FOR YOUR PATHWAY

God's *Pathway to Healing* has six specific principles for identifying your particular *Pathway to Healing* for whatever mountain or attack that you may be facing in your body. Your healing may supernaturally and instantaneously manifest, or you may experience a process that combines His supernatural power with wisdom, taking the specific actions necessary to obtain your healing.

Your *Pathway to Healing* may involve a passage of time in which you will want to both pray and listen carefully to your physical temple, your body. To know what actions God desires you to take, you need to pray with understanding about your particular disease or ailment. The Bible urges us to pray with understanding: "What is it then? I will pray with the spirit, and I will *pray with the understanding* also" (1 Corinthians 14:15, emphasis ours). To pray with understanding, apply these six principles that will reveal your *Pathway to Healing.*

PRINCIPLE 1:
CAST YOUR CARES ON THE LORD

Negative, unhealthy, and destructive emotions like fear, anxiety, and worry can hinder your prayers about whatever disease

you are facing and keep you from understanding what actions the Holy Spirit
wants you to take. First Peter 5:7 AMP
states, "Casting the whole of your care – all
your anxieties, all your worries, all your
concerns, once and for all – on Him; for
He cares for you affectionately, and cares
about you watchfully."

If you are facing worries and fears about
a particular disease, we want to reassure you
that by the stripes of Jesus you have been
healed (see 1 Peter 2:24). We often share
with patients, "You must cast all of your
anxieties and cares upon God. Cast your
worries upon the Lord once and for all!"

We might have a person worried about
a disease pray these words:

*Father, in the name of Jesus I come
before Your throne. You instructed me in
1 Peter 5:7 to cast all of my care, all of*

my worry, and all of my anxiety once and for all upon You. Because You instructed me to do this, I know that I am capable of doing this and being set free of anxiety. So I cast the anxiety I have about [whatever disease you are facing] upon You. You did not give me a spirit of fear, so I cast all of my concern about this problem upon You. I thank You that, according to Psalm 91, I will be satisfied with long life. Amen.

We will also instruct a person that fear may well attack again in a day or so after we have prayed. We then instruct patients not to pray this same prayer about fear again. Instead we explain that the enemy is attacking the mind with fear and we must now take authority over him:

Satan, I have cast any anxiety about [speak your disease here] on my heavenly Father just as He told me to do. He would not tell me to cast my cares upon Him unless it was something I am capable of doing. Therefore, satan, I take authority over you, and I command you to stop attacking my mind with fearful thoughts.

PRINCIPLE 2:
PRAY AND PETITION GOD FOR YOUR PATHWAY TO HEALING

Our key text here is Philippians 4:6-7, "But in every thing by prayer and supplication with thanksgiving let your requests be made known unto God. And the peace of God, which passeth all understanding, shall keep your hearts and minds through Christ Jesus." Pray according to these verses:

Father, I thank You that You will reveal to me the specific pathway that will lead to the healing of all of my symptoms. I thank You, Father, that in Jesus' name I will not experience problems any longer with this ailment such as [list the symptoms you are having here]. I thank You, Father, that You have provided ways to protect my temple through the use of plant derived chemicals. They will protect me from disease and reverse any symptoms present in my body. Let Your healing anointing flow through these substances. Thank You, Father, for granting these petitions in Jesus' name. Amen.

PRINCIPLE 3:
TEST YOUR OPTIONS
BY THE SPIRIT OF GOD

As you seek God for your *Pathway to Healing,* let the Holy Spirit reveal your options and check or stop any choices that He does not desire you to take. The Bible instructs us: "And let the peace (soul harmony which comes) from Christ rule (act as umpire continually) in your hearts [deciding and settling with finality all questions that arise in your minds, in that peaceful state] to which as [members of Christ's] one body you were also called [to live]. And be thankful (appreciative), [giving praise to God always]" (Colossians 3:15 AMP).

The Spirit of God helps us to consider carefully our options – He umpires our choices – until we reach a decision that brings complete peace in our lives. Simply pray:

Father, I pray that the Holy Spirit will act as an umpire in my life according to Colossians 3:15, guiding me to every right decision in Your perfect will for me. Grant me Your peace in each decision that Your Spirit guides me through. In Jesus' name. Amen.

PRINCIPLE 4:
SPEAK TO THE MOUNTAIN

Now you are ready to speak to the mountain. Instead of just praying, petitioning, and testing, you can go even further using the authority that God gave you. Jesus taught us to speak to our mountain and command that mountain (in this case, illness) to be removed. "For verily I say unto you, That whosoever shall say unto this mountain, Be thou removed, and be thou cast into the sea; and shall not doubt in his heart, but shall believe that those things which he saith shall come to pass; he shall have whatsoever he saith" (Mark 11:23). So when you speak to the mountain in prayer, you might pray:

Father, I come before You in Jesus' name and I speak to this mountain called [name the disease or symptom]. I command my body to be normal and I command my body and [name the symptoms] to line up with the Word of God. Thank You, Father, for the power that You have given me through the name of Jesus to speak to my mountain. Thank You, Father, that through that authority I have dominion over the works of darkness that would attack my temple which houses the precious treasure that You placed within me. In Jesus' name I pray. Amen.

Principle 5:
Persist and Stand Firm in Your Pathway

When you have a revelation of God's *Pathway to Healing* for whatever challenge you are facing in your body, stand firm in what He is guiding you to do. "Wherefore take unto you the whole armour of God, that ye may be able to withstand in the evil day, and having done all, to stand" (Ephesians 6:13).

You can stand firm and persist by following a proper nutrition and supplement plan to maintain the correct balance of various chemicals in your body. You must stand firm that as you do all you can do in the natural to protect your temple through nutrition, exercise, and the use of herbs, you will not suffer the ravages of disease affecting the various organs, nerves, and blood vessels in your body.

PRINCIPLE 6:
MAINTAIN A FEISTY ATTITUDE AGAINST THE WORKS OF DARKNESS

In order to persist and stand firm, you must shift to a different attitude. Avoid the danger of becoming passive, giving up, or failing to fight this battle. Be feisty – even violent – in your persistence. "And from the days of John the Baptist until now the kingdom of heaven suffereth violence, and the violent take it by force" (Matthew 11:12).

We encourage you to maintain a feisty attitude against all of the symptoms that are taking place in your body. In God's *Pathway to Healing*, He wants you to be satisfied with a long life. The word satisfied means that you are free of pain and symptoms in your physical body. We know that according to Revelation 22:2, "the leaves of the tree were for the healing of the nations." This scripture can have multiple meanings. One of the meanings is how God *did* use natural substances found in plants to work through to achieve our healing. God will give you clear direction as to what can be of particular help to your own body chemistry as you follow these specific principles. You will even be alerted to things that will not be helpful, or perhaps even harmful, to your body.

Chapter 5

YOUR NEXT STEPS
IN GOD'S *PATHWAY*
TO HEALING

Chapter 5

YOUR NEXT STEPS IN GOD'S *PATHWAY TO HEALING*

You have begun an important journey toward finding your *Pathway to Healing* from whatever you might be battling in your body. Act on the truths you have received from God.

We want to review and summarize for you the steps you need to take now as you receive God's unique *Pathway to Healing* for you.

Step 1. Consult with a physician. Consultation with a physician or a competent medical person can give you information about your body and give you particular insight as to how to pray for your symptoms. Even better is a Christian physician who will pray the prayer of agreement with you. A physician can also alert you to potential dangers of herbs and possible interactions with other substances you are already putting into your body.

Step 2. Pray with understanding. Seek God in prayer. Ask Him to reveal to you and your physician the things you need to do in the natural as you walk down your *Pathway to Healing.*

Step 3. Ask the Holy Spirit to guide you to truth. For example, your doctor may advise you to use a particular medication to treat a symptom or problem in your body. By referring to the information in this book, you can bring up the discussion of certain herbs that have been shown to help with your particular problem. Approach the physician by asking him if he would work with you and try the herbal approach first. Many physicians are open to this approach, even if they are not that familiar with complementary treatments using herbs. Allow the Holy Spirit to guide you and your physician to all truth.

Step 4. Maintain proper and healthy nutrition. Exercise and stay fit. We encourage you to stay on the Mediterranean diet and to use the foods, herbs, and other supplements we have discussed earlier in this book to help your body overcome the symptoms you are battling.

Step 5. Stand firm in *God's Pathway to Healing* **for you.** Refuse to be discouraged or defeated. Be violently aggressive in prayer and in faith, claiming your healing in Jesus Christ.

We are praying that God will both reveal His *Pathway to Healing through Herbs That Heal* to you and give you the strength and faith to walk down this path.

REGINALD B. CHERRY, M.D.

A MEDICAL DOCTOR'S TESTIMONY

The first six years of my life were lived in the dusty, rural town of Mansfield, in the Ouachita Mountains of western Arkansas. In those childhood years, I had one seemingly impossible dream — to be a doctor! Through God's grace, I attended premed at Baylor University and graduated from the University of Texas Medical School in San Antonio, Texas. Throughout those years, I felt God tug on my heart a number of times, especially through Billy Graham as he preached on television. But I never surrendered my life to Jesus Christ.

In those early years of practicing medicine, I met Dr. Kenneth Cooper and was trained in the field of preventive medicine. In the mid-seventies, I moved to Houston and established a medical practice for preventive medicine. Sadly, at that time money became the driving force in my life. Nevertheless, God was good to me. He brought into our clinic a nurse who became a Spirit-filled Christian and she began praying for me. In fact, she had her whole church praying for me!

In my search for fulfillment and meaning in life, I called out to God one night in late November of 1979 and prayed, "Jesus, I give You everything I own. I'm sorry for the life I've lived. I want to live for You the rest of my days. I give You my life." A doctor had been born again. Oh, and by the way, that beautiful nurse who had prayed for me and shared Jesus with me is now my wife, Linda!

Not only did Jesus transform my life; He also transformed my medical practice. God spoke to me and said, " I want you to establish a Christian clinic. From now on when you practice medicine, you will be *ministering* to patients." I began to pray for patients seeking God's *Pathway to Healing* in the supernatural realm as well as in the natural realm.

Over the years, we have witnessed how God has miraculously used both supernatural and natural pathways to heal our patients and to demonstrate His marvelous healing and saving power.

I know what God has done in my life, and I know what God has done in the lives of our patients. He can do the same in your life! He has a unique *Pathway to Healing* for you! He is the Lord who heals you (see Exodus 15:26), and by His stripes you were healed (see Isaiah 53:5).

Know that Linda and I are standing with you as you seek *God's Pathway to Healing: Herbs That Heal,* and as you walk in His *Pathway to Healing* for your life. If you do not know Jesus Christ as your personal Lord and Savior, I invite you to pray this prayer and ask Jesus into your life:

Lord Jesus, I invite You into my life as my Lord and Savior. I turn away from my past sins. I ask You to forgive me. Thank You for shedding Your blood on the cross to cleanse me from my sins and to bring healing to my body. I receive Your gift of everlasting life and surrender all to You. Thank You, Jesus, for saving me. Amen.

ABOUT THE AUTHOR

Reginald B. Cherry, M.D., did his premed at Baylor University, graduated from the University of Texas Medical School, and practiced diagnostic and preventive medicine for over 25 years. His work in medicine has been recognized and honored by the city of Houston and by the governor of Texas, George W. Bush. Dr. Cherry's wife, Linda, is a clinical nurse and has worked with Dr. Cherry with patients during these 25 years. Dr. Cherry and Linda also appear weekly on their television program, *"The Doctor and the Word,"* which goes into over 100 million households. Dr. Cherry speaks and lectures extensively and his first two books, *The Doctor and the Word* and *The Bible Cure,* each have made the best sellers' list.

RESOURCES AVAILABLE THROUGH REGINALD B. CHERRY MINISTRIES, INC.

The Bible Cure — Dr. Cherry presents truths hidden in the Bible taken from ancient dietary health laws, how Jesus anointed natural substances to heal, and how to activate faith through prayer for health and healing. This book validates scientific medical research by proving God's original health plan.

$16.99 + S&H

The Doctor and The Word — (now in paperback) Dr. Cherry introduces how God has a *Pathway to Healing* for you. Jesus healed both instantaneously and supernaturally while other healings involved a process. Discover how the manifestation of your healing can come about by seeking His ways. $10.99 + S&H

God's Pathway to Healing: **Menopause** — This minibook is full of helpful advice for women who are going through what can be a very stressful time of life. Find out what foods, supplements, and steps can be taken to find a *Pathway to Healing* for menopause and perimenopause.

$10.00 + S&H

Pathway to Healing Seminar — Listen to Dr. Cherry and Linda as they teach before a live audience at Lakewood Church. Walk down your *Pathway to Healing* as you discover how to protect your temple which contains the Holy Spirit. (8 tapes) $29.99 + S&H

Bound Volume of Study Guides — Receive 35 valuable resource study guides from topics Dr. Cherry has taught on television over the past twelve years — cancer, vitamins, the immune system, weight loss, chronic fatigue, arthritis, nutrition, diabetes, and many other subjects.

$20.00 + S&H

BECOME A *PATHWAY TO HEALING* PARTNER

We invite you to become a **Pathway Partner.** We ask you to stand with us in prayer and financial support as we provide new programs, new resources, new books, minibooks, and a unique, one-of-a-kind monthly newsletter.

Our monthly *Pathway to Healing* **Partner Newsletter** is packed with medical and biblical information that only Pathway Partners receive. Here are the features our newsletter contains:

Dr. Cherry's Personal Letter — A front-page letter each month brimming with the latest medical information and biblical revelation on your *Pathway to Healing*.

Fearfully & Wonderfully Made (Psalm 139:14) — Medical science is continually discovering what Scripture already reveals — that our bodies are miraculous creations given to us by God. In this feature, Dr. Cherry shares startling facts about our temples (how doctors diagnose thyroid disease by looking at the eyebrows, for example) and how God designed our immune system, hormones, arteries, kidneys, etc. to work in balance the way God "made" us.

Ask Dr. Cherry: Your Questions Are Answered (Luke 11:5-10) — Read Dr. Cherry's direct responses each month to your specific questions. We want to provide you with both clear instruction and precise information by answering your questions as space permits.

I Will Allow None of These Diseases on You (Exodus 15:26) —This monthly feature uncovers what the Bible teaches about God's healing at work in your temple. Discover how to pray specifically and biblically for your health concerns.

Praying With Understanding (1 Corinthians 14:15) — Dr. Cherry teaches you how to pray specifically for diseases, healing, and removing mountains from your life. There are prayers that Dr. Cherry and Linda have prayed personally with patients to remove their mountains of heart disease, cancer, diabetes, hypertension, arthritis, worry, depression, and other afflictions that attack our temples. The more you understand how to pray about a problem and how to speak to your mountain (Mark 11:23), the more effective your prayer will be (James 5:16).

Good Reports Give Happiness & Health (Proverbs 15:30) — We share good reports from our Partners of what God is doing to give you hope. The reports are intended to give all the glory to God. Be encouraged as you read what God is doing to "satisfy you with long life."

Nutrition & Your Health (Genesis 1:29) — God has created plants, herbs, minerals, and certain proteins for you to consume for energy and for strengthening your immune system, which prevents and overcomes disease. Through proper nutrition, you can stay healthy! Learn what to eat, how to exercise, what supplements fight disease, and how to maintain a proper balance of nutrition in your *Pathway to Healing*.

Linda's Kitchen (Exodus 23:25) — Linda's recipes are filled with good nutrition and will teach you how to eat healthy according to God's *Bible Cure*. They are based on the wealth of knowledge gleaned from the Levitical dietary laws and wisdom revealed in Scripture about how to take care of our bodies. Read about how she cooks at home using her actual recipes.

In addition, we'll provide you with Dr. Cherry & Linda's ministry calendar, broadcast schedule, resources for better living, and special monthly offers.

Call or write to the address below to obtain information on how you can receive this valuable resource.

Pathway to Healing **Partner Newsletter** — Available to you as you partner with Dr. Cherry's ministry through prayer and monthly financial support to help expand this God-given ministry. Pray today about responding. Contribution of $10.00 or more monthly.

Become a Pathway Partner today by
calling toll-free:
1 - 888 – DrCherry
(1 – 888 - 372 - 4377)

Or writing:
Reginald B. Cherry Ministries, Inc.
P. O. Box 27711
Houston, TX 77227

Visit our website:
www.drcherry.org

BOOKS BY
REGINALD B. CHERRY, M.D.

God's Pathway to Healing:

Menopause

God's Pathway to Healing:

Herbs that Heal

Additional copies of this book and other book titles
from ALBURY PUBLISHING are
available at your local bookstore.

ALBURY PUBLISHING
Tulsa, Oklahoma 74147-0406

For a complete list of our titles,
visit us at our website:
www.alburypublishing.com

For international and Canadian orders,
please contact:

Access Sales International
2448 East 81st Street
Suite 4900
Tulsa, Oklahoma 74137
Phone 918-523-5590 Fax 918-496-2822